The first day without sunshine

Written By J.R. Denney

Illustrated By Phillipa Haskins

The First Day Without Sunshine

© 2021 J.R. Denney

Illustrations © Phillipa Haskins

For my sunbeam, Brandi.

The sun is the center of our world.

It is our light.

Beaming out of the sun is our

sunshine.

Our sunshine is the people or things that we love and love us.

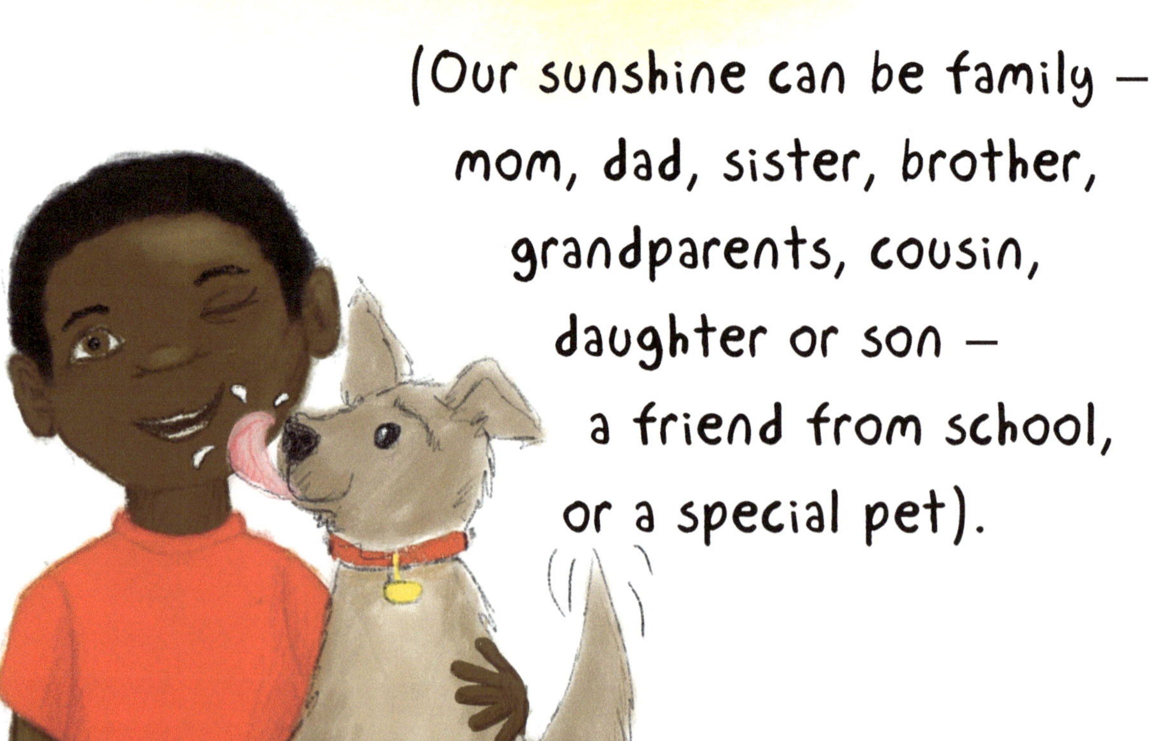

(Our sunshine can be family —
mom, dad, sister, brother,
grandparents, cousin,
daughter or son —
a friend from school,
or a special pet).

Your sunshine can be almost anything.
It is the part of the sun that touches you and is made up of sunbeams, the people or things in our lives that fill us with love and hope in good times and bad.

Our sunshine shines down on us from the sun, on everything that we love, **big** or small.

But our special sunbeams
don't always last forever.

Sometimes those sunbeams go away.

They leave

or die

or neglect you.

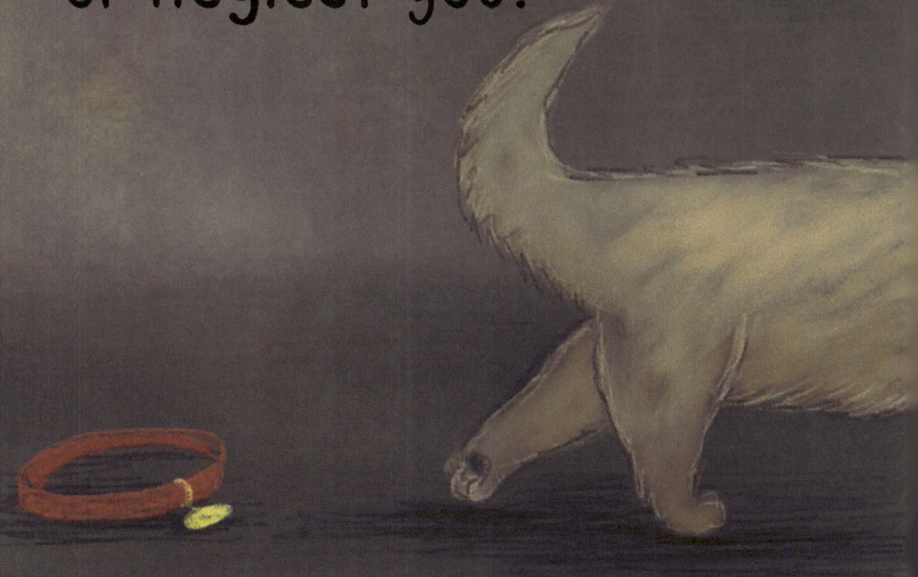

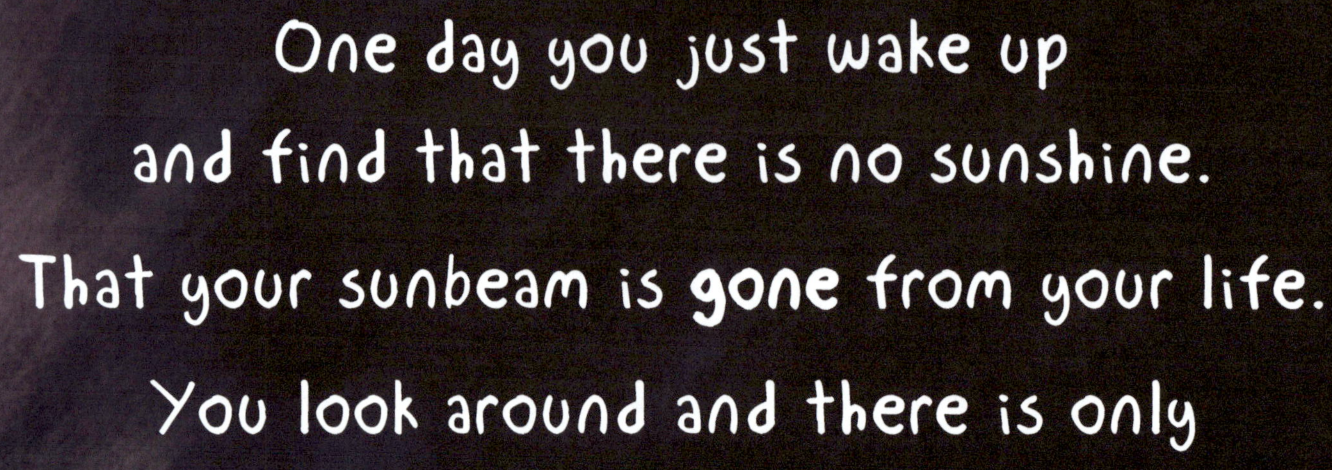

One day you just wake up
and find that there is no sunshine.

That your sunbeam is **gone** from your life.

You look around and there is only

darkness.

You are upset
and scared,
and it makes you feel so bad
that it hurts all over.

You try to pretend that it's not true,
that it is not really happening,
that it must be a dream,
and all you have to do

is wake up.

The sunbeam that you love so much
can't really be gone,

they couldn't have left,
they just couldn't.

This is natural.

It is just the way we feel.

It's normal to not believe
that your sunshine is gone.

Most of the time,
this is the first thing that we feel.

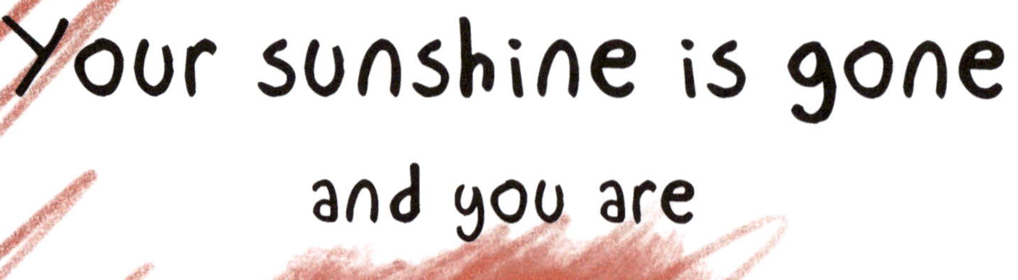

Your sunshine is gone
and you are

angry

and **hurt,**

or feel **guilty**

or **even mad**

at the sun
and the other sunbeams.

You may need to cry
or to be held

or maybe just need
for someone
to sit down on the
ground beside you.

But at the same time,
all you want is for the sun
and the other sunbeams
to go away
and leave you
alone
because you don't want to be touched
by the sun
or the other sunbeams in your life.

It isn't fair that your
special sunbeam
is gone.

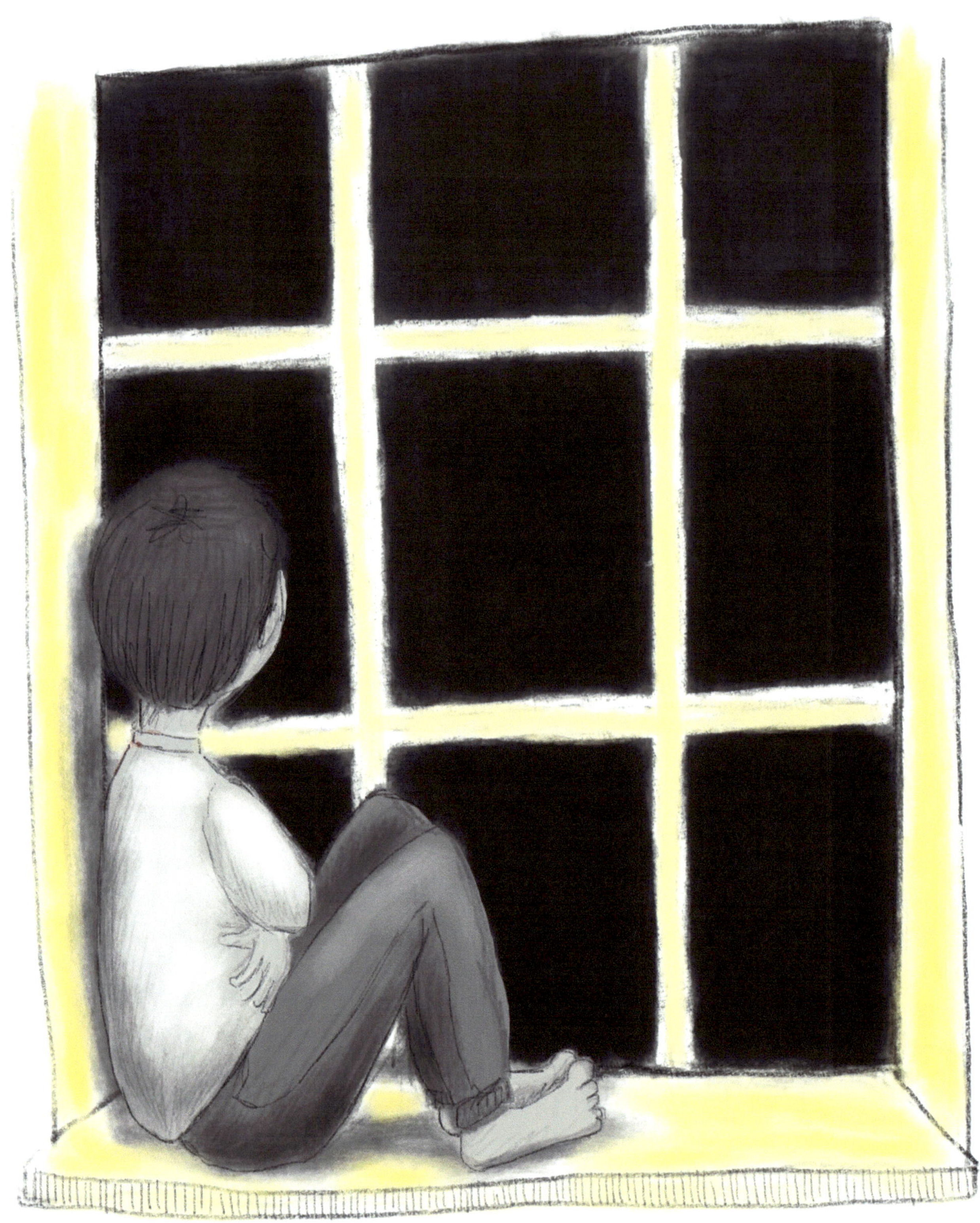

This is natural.

Most of the time,
anger is the second thing that we feel
when we realize our sunbeam is gone.

We hurt so bad
it makes us ache all over,

and no matter what anyone says or does,
it just will not stop

or go away.

It isn't fair your sunbeam is gone
and the sun is cold and dark.

So, you cry
or you beg
for your sunbeam
to come home.

You try to figure out what it
was that you did to cause this.

You even try talk God
into helping you out.

You offer to do anything,
make any bargain
to get your sunbeam back.

You give your word
that you will change,
that you will be good.

You pledge that you
will pay attention,
and vow to quit doing
whatever it was that you believe
you might have done to cause this.

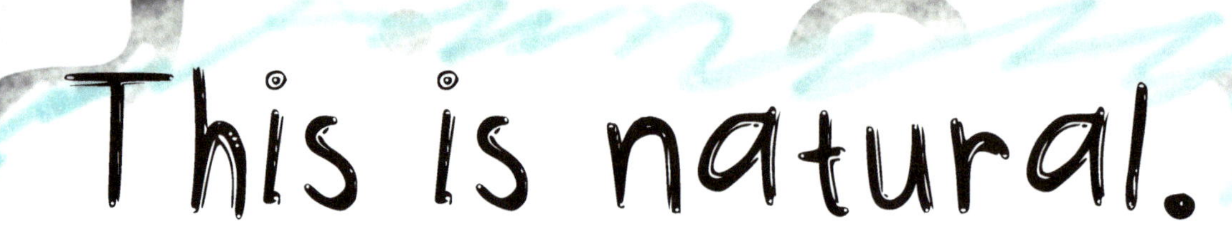

This is natural.

We blame ourselves.

We bargain.

We believe that we must have done **something wrong** to deserve this.

That it is our punishment.

It is not a punishment.

You didn't do anything wrong, sometimes bad things just happen.

It is natural to **blame** and to try to **bargain**.

It is what we often feel after anger.

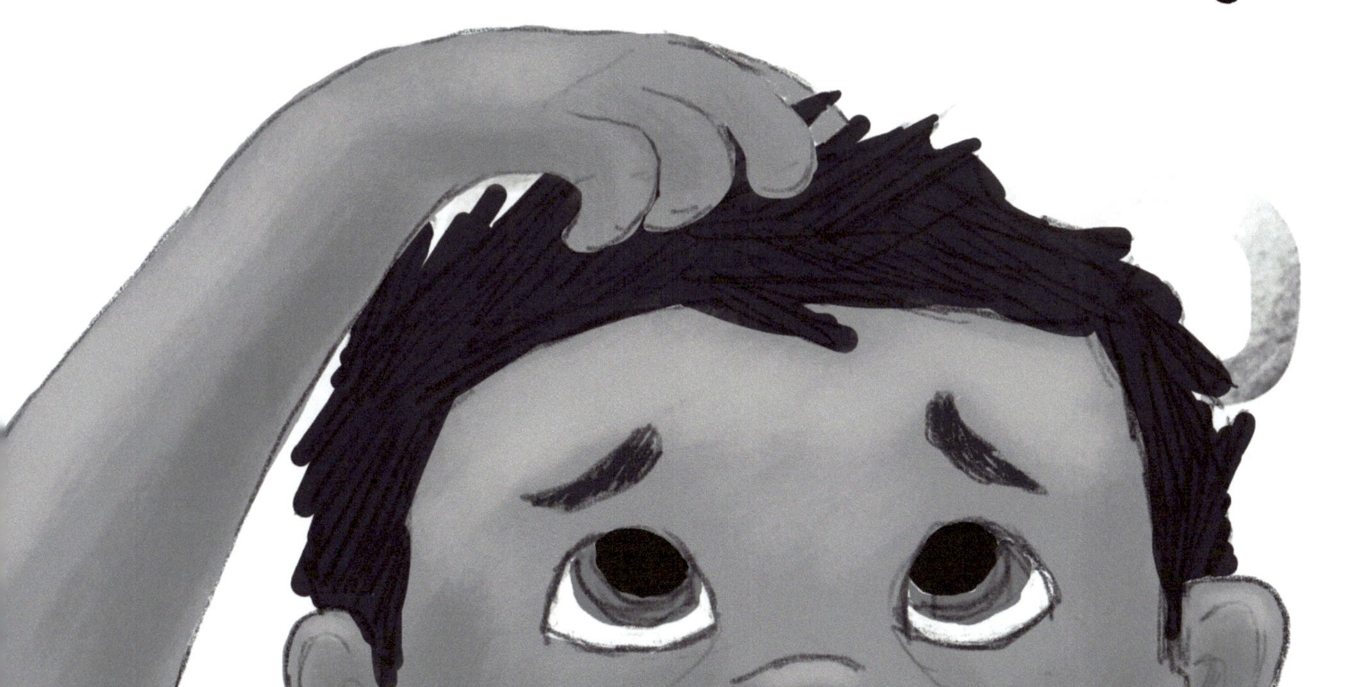

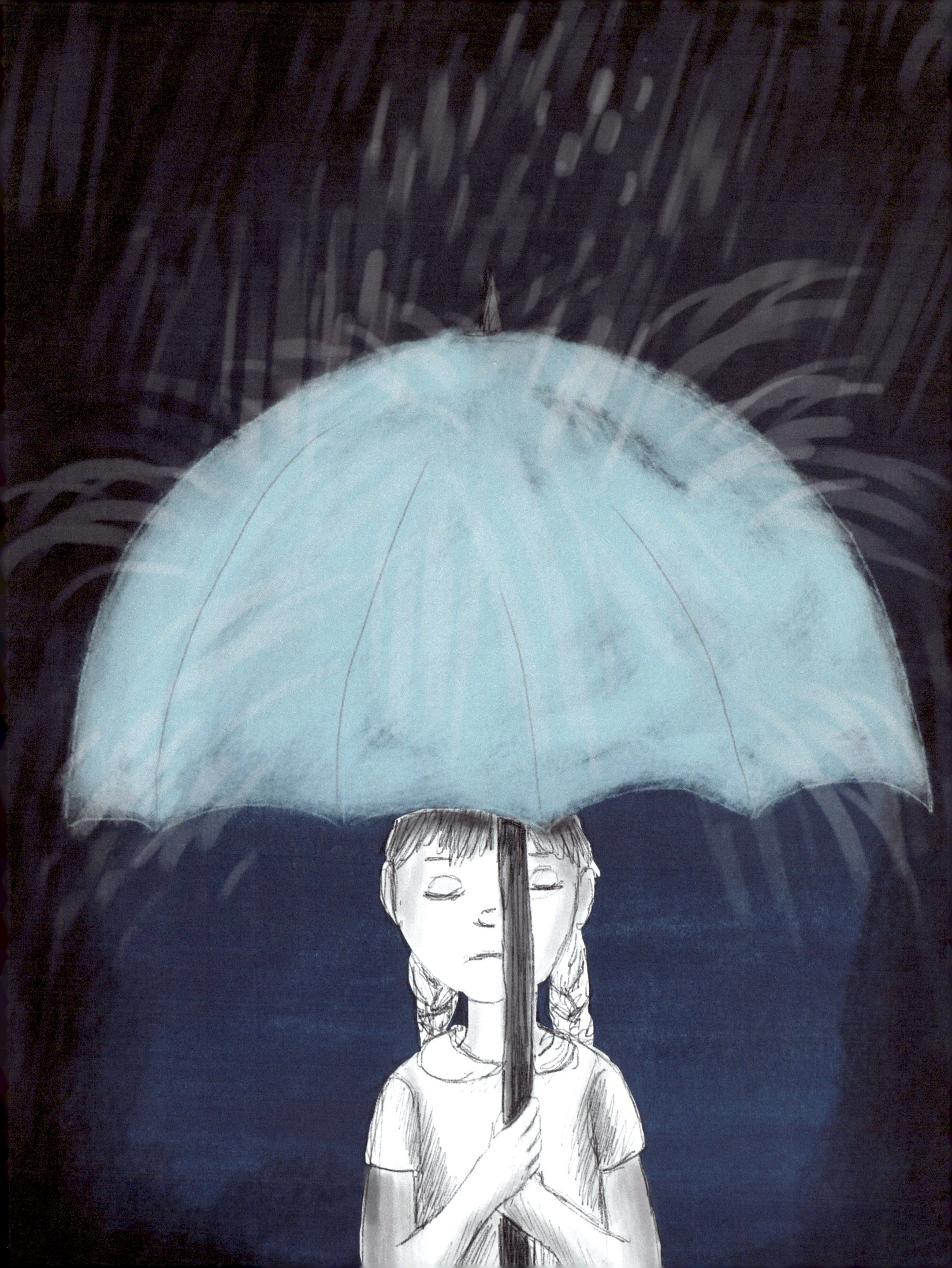

Then, after **disbelief**
and **anger**
and **blame,**
comes the time when you look around
and realize that your sunbeam
isn't coming back.

Your sun has **changed forever.**

It is darker.

It is clouded and gray with grief.

It makes you hurt all over.
It might even hurt so bad that it makes you
sick.

You don't want to do the things
that you used to do,
you're **heartbroken** and **lonely,**
feeling **sad** and **depressed.**

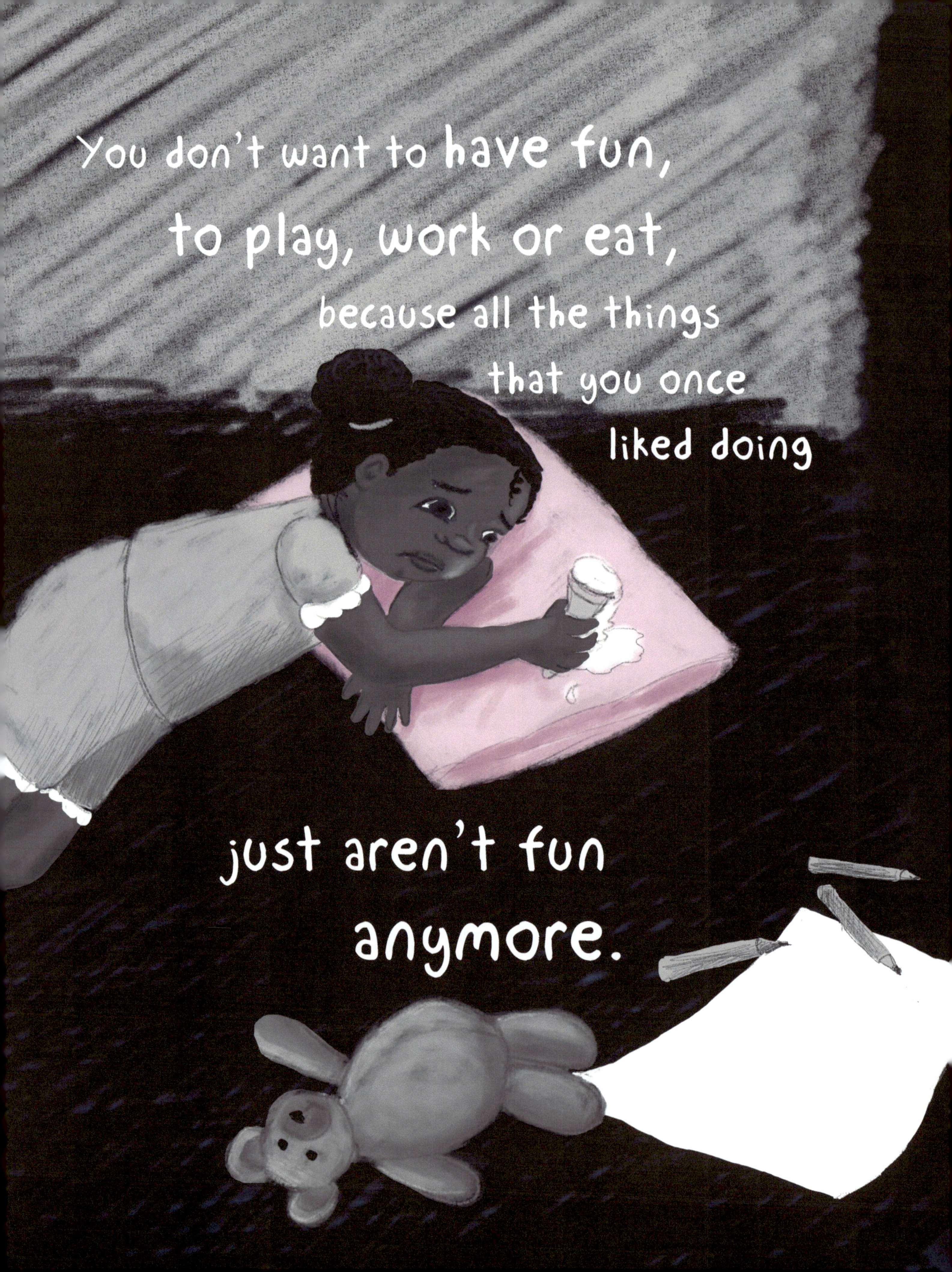

You don't want to have fun,
to play, work or eat,
because all the things
that you once
liked doing

just aren't fun
anymore.

This is natural.

Feeling sad and depressed
after you lose something that you love
is normal.
It is usually the fourth thing that you'll feel.

Most of the time,
sadness will visit you
after you finally realize
that your sunbeam isn't coming back,
and before you are able to
accept it
in your heart.

Then,
finally,
one day you wake up
and you realize that there is

still light

coming through your window.

It's not as bright
as it once was,
or as happy,
but it is sunshine
carried on other

sunbeams

who
have
been
there
all
along.

You just
didn't see them.

You realize

there was nothing

that you did

or could have done

to change anything that happened,

and that your sunbeam

probably wouldn't want

you to remember them

that way anyways.

Your sunbeam would want you
to remember them as

loving
and
happy.

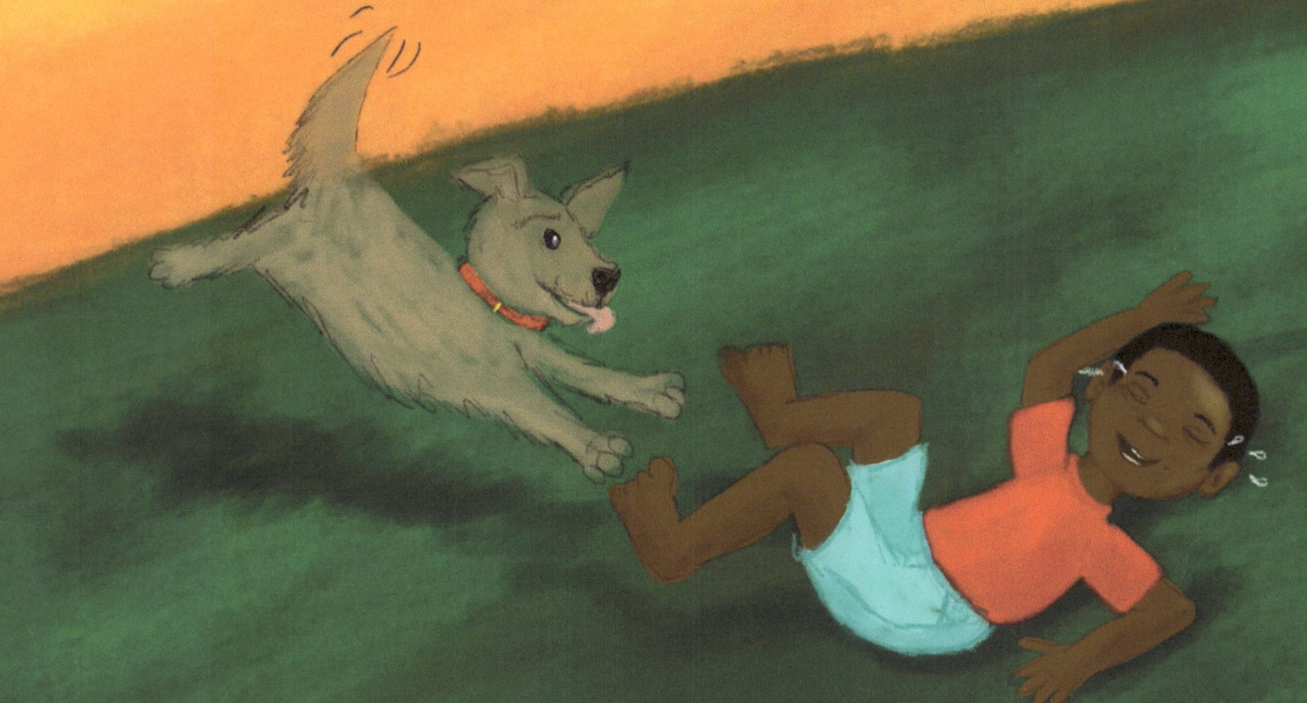

They would want you
to remember
the funny times you shared.

And,
most of all,
for you to remember
that they were

your special

sunbeam,
and that as long
as you keep them
in your heart,

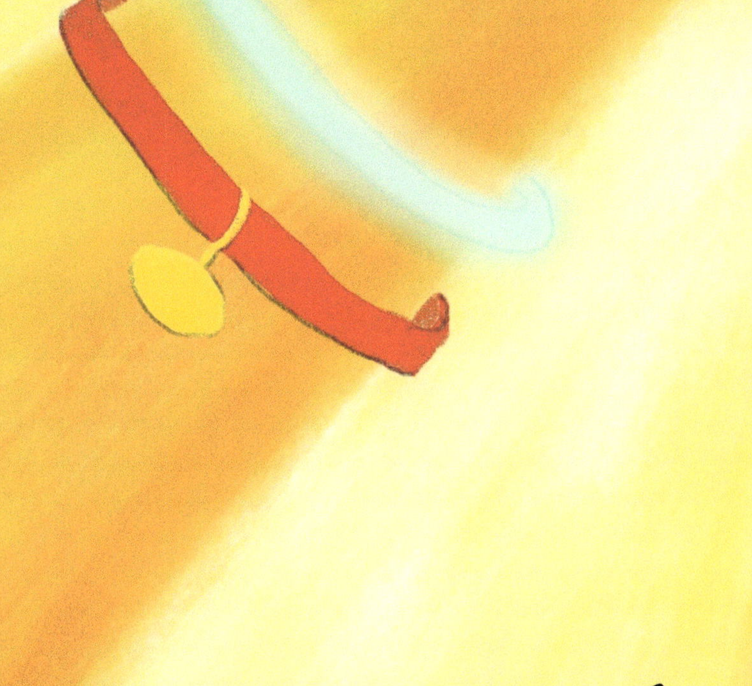

they are not
really gone at all.

www.ingramcontent.com/pod-product-compliance
Lightning Source LLC
Chambersburg PA
CBHW041136260726
48664CB00027B/1224